THE BEGINNER'S GUIDE TO MACROS & FLEXIBLE DIETING

BY IFBB BIKINI PRO
CHRISTINA FRISCIA

DEDICATION:

To the woman who has struggled with her body image, with listening to a thousand voices and opinions, with allowing judgement from others to influence how she feels about herself. The next time you want to talk bad about yourself, think about saying those things to the 6 year old version of you, and please remember just how beautiful, strong, powerful, and worthy you are, just as you are. I love you, I see you, I am you.

CONTENTS

CHRISTINA FRISCIA

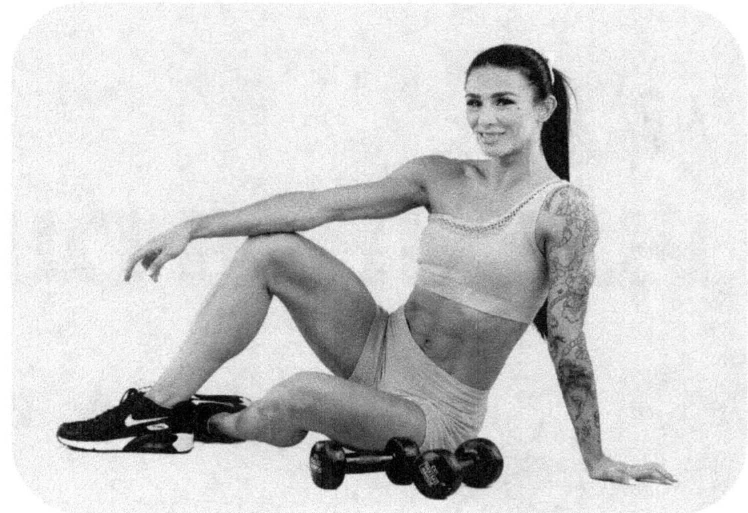

INTRODUCTION

Hey babe! Thanks so much for buying The Beginner's Guide to Macros & Flexible Dieting! This was designed to help you learn the in's and out's of flexible/macro based dieting, including how to actually calculate your own macros, how to track them within your meals, and how to finally achieve those physique goals that seemed to never happen previously, no matter what you've tried or done.

The beauty of flexible dieting is this:

IT'S NOT A TREND

This system and these calculations will work and be the same for the rest of your life. So, let me ask, what if you never needed to buy a new dieting plan ever again? Or never needed to go through the extreme highs and lows of weight loss, and could actually eat the foods you've come to love without restricting your taste buds & brain of any sort of enjoyment or sensation? What if I told you, you had to hold yourself accountable, but if you did, you'd be off to the races in no time at all? ***Would you be interested in giving it a shot?***

So many people say they're willing to "do anything" to lose the weight, to get in better shape, to feel healthier and more invigorated, but it seems that all they're really willing to do is the extremes. Enough of the extreme measures. **What you really need is to do the basics consistently and well. Let's get started...**

What is
FLEXIBLE DIETING?

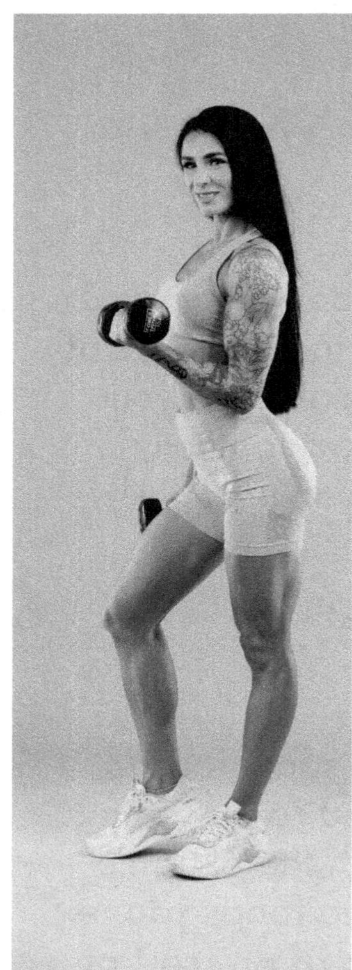

The solution to your dieting woes...

When it comes to counting macros, the beauty is in the flexibility of the plan. Flexible dieting is a popular and simple weight loss program that allows you to eat any foods you like, so long as they fit within your specific daily macronutrient targets. This way of eating and viewing nutrition provides you freedom in your food choices, which may help keep weight off over time and create a better, more positive and healthy relationship with food.

Plus, it's very easy to stick to, no matter if you're eating at home or on the go. The days of not being able to eat out or enjoy family time because you're "on a diet" are over! That's no way to live and totally unnecessary today.

The problem some people find themselves in and why flexible dieting tends to get a bad rap is because although you have the freedom to fill your macros with the foods you desire, it's still your responsibility to make sure you're eating whole, healthy foods regularly, and not filling your macros with Pop Tarts and Oreos, with very little fiber or nutritional value seen. So although flexible dieting is a wonderful tool to learn how to eat freely while still going after your physique goals, you still need to be responsible and smart.

We know that preparation is the key to success...

But how often do you find yourself scrambling to put something together for dinner, or just saying SCREW IT and ordering take out? If it's more than once a week, you're overdue for a routine change!

Meal prepping and tracking your food go together hand in hand with flexible dieting. The most success I've ever found with my own journey and with my clients was when the meals were tracked and planned well ahead of time, and not left to the last minute. When you attack your nutrition meal by meal, what inevitably happens is, you're left at the end of the night with a chunk of random macros to fill, and no idea what to eat to fix it. So, you either go over your macros and feel guilty, or, you say, "forget it, I'll try again tomorrow." and you go to bed without eating enough. Put it this way, you're given $1000 to go on a shopping spree, but you only spend $818 of it, then say "I don't want the rest." Doesn't make sense, right? Well, that's what you're doing to your macros and nutrition when you don't eat to your goals. What's the point of having goals if you're going to leave them hanging?

We've been taught since we're children that eating less will make us lose weight. *But if only it were really that simple.* The problem with this mindset is that metabolic adaptations happen very quickly, and when your body get too used to eating lower amounts than it requires, it has no option but to survive on the lower calories, and your fat/weight loss and muscle gain will suffer as a result.

Why does your body stop losing weight when food is too low?

Our bodies were designed to survive and keep us alive, not to change/grow muscle/lose weight. So we need to counteract these primitive systems our bodies tend to default to when we're trying to get in shape. When calories get too low and expenditure gets too high, your body & brain don't know the difference between you just trying to get in shape vs. you starving in the middle of the jungle. **All it knows is it's not receiving enough sustenance to keep you going, so it protects you by holding onto body fat and water, and refusing to build muscle AKA SURVIVAL MODE!**

Fast Facts to Remember
MACROS

Macros stands for macronutrients.
Macronutrients are the nutritive components of food that the body needs for energy and to maintain the body's structure and systems. *Carbohydrates, Fat and Protein* are your macronutrients. They are the nutrients you use in the largest amounts. Fiber & water are also sometimes considered macronutrients, but for the sake of flexible dieting, we typically track the Big 3.

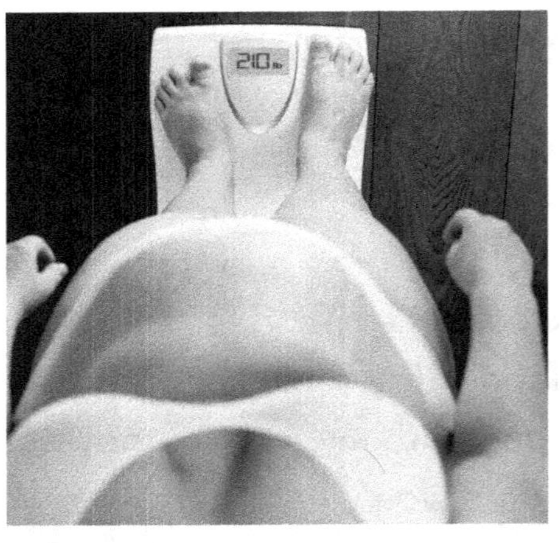

Anyone can work out for an hour. True strength is controlling what goes on your plate during the other 23...

For quick notation, please remember:
Each gram of **carbohydrates** is **4 calories.**
Each gram of **protein** is **4 calories.**
Each gram of **fat** is **9 calories.**
1 LB = 3500 Calories
Ideal weight loss/gain goal= 1-2lbs per week max
(Any more than that will start to impede skin elasticity and hormones.)

Your daily caloric goal is where we start, and from that number, we are then able to break it down into an ideal macro split. Let's get to the calculations next.

How to Create Your Macro Split?
Step 1: Calculating BMR

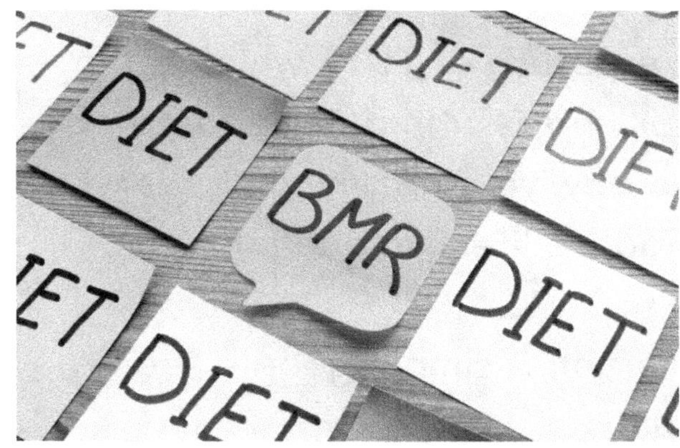

Before we can determine your ideal calories and macro split, we need to determine your **BASAL METABOLIC RATE aka BMR**. This is basically the amount of calories your body requires just to stay alive and keep all basic human functions (like brain health, keeping your blood flowing and heart pumping, etc) active and optimal.

There are BMR calculators available for you to use all over the internet, so you can find one to do the calculations for you.

But, if you prefer to do it the old school way, you will want to use the following calculation. This is also known as the **Harris-Benedict Formula.**

For Men:

66.5 + (13.75 x Weight in kg) + (5.003 x Height in cm) – (6.755 x age in years)

For Women:

655.1 + (9.563 x weight in kg) + (1.850 x height in cm) – (4.676 x age in years)

How to Create Your Macro Split?
Step 2: Calculating TDEE

After you find out your BMR, you'll then need to factor in activity calories!

This is also called your **Total Daily Energy Expenditure or TDEE** which is the total number of calories your body uses on a daily basis with activity factored into it. If you are more sedentary throughout the day, your activity calories will be much less than someone with a very active lifestyle and job.

TDEE calculators are also found all over the internet. A simple google search can give you many options.

But for quick reference, here is how those numbers are calculated.

To find your TDEE, use the following equation:
SEDENTARY (Little to no exercise) : BMR x 1.2
LIGHTLY ACTIVE (Light exercise/sports 3-5x per week): BMR x 1.375
MODERATELY ACTIVE (Moderate exercise/sports 3-5x per week): BMR x 1.55
VERY ACTIVE (Hard exercise/sports 6-7x per week): BMR x 1.725
EXTRA ACTIVE (Hard exercise/sports 6-7x per week + Physical job): BMR x 1.9

This calculation will give you your current "ideal" calories to **maintain** your weight based on where you are right now in terms of activity level. *Keep this number somewhere where you can easily access it.* You will be needing it soon as we move along to the next step. But before we jump into creating your macro split from your TDEE calculated calories, we need to talk about something very important first... **YOUR DIETING HISTORY.**

Why Your Previous Dieting History Matters!

I mentioned earlier that your body was not designed to constant fluctuate in weight, so it adapts to what you're throwing it very easily. This is a large reason why those who have been living "on a diet" and heavily restricting their calories more often than not are the same people who are always struggling to see any real progress or fat loss. **Because you're being a savage in the worst way possible, and your body is fed up with your shit. Sorry but this is the unfortunate truth.**

Your previous dieting history, whether that be previous eating disorders, gastric surgeries, or you just restricting your intake severely for months or years at a time/being afraid to eat because you don't want to "get fat", is absolutely going to affect your ability to see progress today, even if you're doing everything "right" in your mind. When you've forced your body to live in "survival mode" for extended periods of time, all you can do to get yourself on the other side of the stubbornness and resistance within your metabolism is to literally eat your way out of the hole you've dug yourself into. Sounds scary, I understand. But that fear of food hasn't served you yet, so why not try something different?

Now, I already know what you're thinking. You've been afraid of eating for as long as you can remember. And now I'm telling you that in order to lose fat, you need to eat more. WTF?!

Well, remember how I talked about metabolic adaptations? So, with the amount of restrictions and the frequency, your body has had no choice but to adapt to these low calories and survive on what you've given it. So that diet that might've worked awesome the first time is not going to be enough to give you the same results twice because, like I said, **METABOLIC ADAPTATIONS**.

How to Create Your Macro Split?
STEP 3: Starting a Recomp

Okay, so you calculated your BMR and TDEE numbers, and now that I mentioned possible metabolic adaptations, you're nervous and a bit overwhelmed. It's totally OK. I'm going to help you clear things up.

If you are someone who has been dealing with any of the issues mentioned previously, the next step is to start a RECOMP, also know as the process of changing your body composition. Remember, there are levels to truly mastering this process and also keep in mind, this isn't a diet. This is changing the way you view food for the better for life. So by changing your body composition, weight and fat loss is often the goal as well. But we can't know what your fat loss calories should be until we learn how your body responds to actually tracking average numbers consistently. My goal is not to restrict you long term. Both of our goals should be to rediscover the control you actually have over your body composition and change it in the direction you choose.

So let's start by being consistent with tracking our foods for a period of 4 weeks based on the number you calculated as your TDEE. You might feel frustrated in the beginning and want to give up. You might feel like you're eating too much. But by giving up you're just delaying the inevitable and perpetuating the issues that have plagued you for so long. The goal here is to get your body used to a new normal, and adapt to a healthier caloric intake. By doing this, once we start cutting calories back a bit, the cutting will actually have an effect on body fat and weight loss. Also keep in mind that the majority of women aren't overweight, they're **UNDER MUSCLED.**

So if you can, starting some form of resistance/weight training 3-4x a week can greatly benefit your progress.

Something to note is that the more muscle your body holds, the more food you can eat. Because muscle takes a heck of a lot of food to keep it on your bones. And please, don't fear getting too big too fast. You won't. Unless you're eating like a male bodybuilder and taking steroids for muscle growth. Growing muscle tissue takes a lot of time and effort. I always hear that woman telling me "I don't want to look like a man" and honey, you couldn't look like a man even if you tried. I would never let you lose your femininity. All I want for you is for you to trust yourself, trust me, and trust the process. Allow your body to be fed, and learn to release the guilt that comes with eating.

By starting this recomp, you will soon realize how much better you feel, both mentally and physically, on a day to day basis. Your energy will return, your mood will be more balanced and reliable, and your friends and family will want to know what you're doing differently, because you're glowing.

Just tell them you finally started taking CARE instead of being CONCERNED.

During this time, we are not going to focus on weighing ourselves everyday. We are not going to obsess over the numbers on the scale. We are going to go off of how we feel. You will weigh yourself once per week on your check-in day. (Always first thing in the morning after you use the bathroom and before you eat anything, wear the same outfit or lack there of weekly for consistency.) You should also be taking your measurements once per week on the same day and time. You also want to take progress photos during this time as well, even if they make you uncomfortable. This is simply between you and God. We take progress photos because not even point of progress can be seen on the scale or numbers. But that doesn't mean that your body isn't changing shape. This is why I ask you to take these 3 data points so over time, you can track your progress and stop stressing over just what you see on the scale.

Over these next few weeks, also prepare for fluctuations in both directions. Remember, you threw your body into fight or flight mode for years. It needs time to balance itself back out.

Depending on your starting point, there are a few things that you can anticipate happening during this recomp phase:

1. If you are overweight and have knowingly been overeating consistently, this recomp phase will bring about fat and weight loss.
2.   If you are overweight but have been restricting your food intake for quite some time, this recomp phase will start the process of fat loss by regulating your metabolism to a healthier, more sustainable caloric intake level, likely resulting in fat and weight loss as well.
3. If you have been undereating and trying to gain weight, this time period will allow your body to start to learn how to eat properly and gain weight at a healthy pace without binging or bulking.
4.   If you have been at a weight you're happy with but you just don't love how you look or how your body distributes fat, this period will change your body composition and allow your shape to start taking form, so long as you've bee weight training to build muscle.

Building muscle in the gym is what gives our body the shape we want, not conveniently placed body fat. We want the skin to appear beautiful and smooth, and unfortuantely when we rely on our body's fat deposits to be what gives our legs and glutes shape, we also wind up with cellulite- something many women don't desire. Now, there is nothing wrong with cellulite, as it is a natural response to having fat on our body. But if it is something you don't love to see, this process can and will start to smooth our those areas by building up the muscle density that lies beneath the skin, allowing the muscle tissue to press against the skin tighter and creating a smoother look. Losing body fat also is part of this process.

Remember, the goal isn't always weight loss. It's typically fat loss and muscle gain. This may also mean your weight stays consistent for a period of time, but if you're looking and feeling better, your clothes feel and look better, and you are eating enough without starving yourself or overeating, then how much you weigh really doesn't matter. In fact, unless you are at a weight that is teetering on unhealthy, your weight really shouldn't matter at all.

Calculating Grams of PROTEIN

OKAY! Congratulations, we got through the necessary evils of this process. Are you discouraged or amped up to succeed? That is up to you. But I hope I have at least helped bring some awareness to your situation and helped you start to realize why your previous efforts may not have been working for you.

So you're starting in your recomp phase. You've calculated your daily TDEE. Now, how do we turn this caloric number into your daily macros?

Well, let's start by breaking down what MACROS are again and how they work with your daily calories.
For quick notation, please remember:
Each gram of **<u>PROTEIN</u>** is 4 calories.
Each gram of **<u>CARBOHYDRATES</u>** is 4 calories.
Each gram of **<u>FAT</u>** is 9 calories.

Let's start with a simple example:
Say your daily caloric number you've calculated is 2000 calories per day. Great! But how do you break this number down into how many grams of protein, carbs and fats you have to eat per day?

We will start with our **protein** number.
Proteins are essential macronutrients that play numerous vital roles in a woman's body and nutrition.
Here are some important functions of proteins:

<u>**Muscle Structure and Function:**</u> Proteins are the building blocks of muscles. Adequate protein intake supports muscle growth, repair, and maintenance. This is especially important for individuals engaged in regular physical activity and resistance training.

Calculating Grams of PROTEIN

<u>Enzymes and Metabolic Reactions:</u> Many enzymes that facilitate metabolic reactions are proteins. Enzymes play a crucial role in various physiological processes, including digestion, energy production, and the synthesis of essential molecules.

<u>Hormone Production:</u> Some hormones, such as insulin, glucagon, and growth hormone, are proteins. Hormones are signaling molecules that regulate numerous physiological functions, including metabolism, growth, and reproductive processes.

<u>Immune System Function:</u> Antibodies, which are key components of the immune system, are proteins. They help recognize and neutralize foreign substances like viruses and bacteria.

<u>Transportation of Molecules:</u> Proteins serve as carriers, transporting molecules like oxygen (hemoglobin) and lipids (lipoproteins) throughout the body.

<u>Structural Support:</u> Proteins contribute to the structural integrity of various tissues and organs. Collagen, for example, is a protein that provides strength and structure to connective tissues, including skin, tendons, and ligaments.

<u>Fluid Balance:</u> Proteins help maintain fluid balance in the body by exerting osmotic pressure in the blood vessels, preventing excessive fluid leakage into tissues.

<u>pH Regulation:</u> Proteins act as buffers, helping to regulate the body's pH and maintain a stable internal environment.

Calculating Grams of PROTEIN

<u>Neurotransmitter Synthesis:</u> Some neurotransmitters, which are chemical messengers in the nervous system, are synthesized from amino acids, the building blocks of proteins.

<u>Cellular Repair and Maintenance:</u> Proteins are essential for repairing and replacing damaged cells. This process is ongoing and crucial for overall health and longevity.

The recommended dietary allowance (RDA) for protein intake varies depending on factors such as age, activity level, and health status. ***Generally, the RDA for protein for most adults is 1 grams of protein per pound of body weight.*** However, individuals engaged in intense physical activity or those with specific health conditions may require higher protein intake. It's essential to include a variety of protein sources in the diet, such as lean meats, poultry, fish, eggs, dairy products, legumes, nuts, and seeds.

So if you are 150 lbs, you want to eat 150 grams of protein per day.

<u>So let's do that quick math:</u>

150 grams x 4 calories per gram= 600 calories per day of protein
2000 calories per day – 600 calories from protein = 1400 calories remaining

Cool, now we have 1400 calories left to play with...
This is where the flexibility comes into play a bit, and where you can start to have a bit more fun with your food and meals to achieve the same goal calorically, but by varying your food options to fit your desires and needs.

Calculating Grams of FAT

We will get into actually tracking our food in a future section. But for now, let's determine your next number: **FAT GOALS.**

Fat is a crucial part of nutrition, and the word itself has such a negative connotation that it actually infuriates me. None of us are FAT. We just *have* fat. That's healthy, natural, and **NECESSARY**.

Fat plays several important roles in a woman's health. It's crucial to recognize that not all fats are created equal, and different types of fats have distinct effects on health.

Here's an overview of the roles of fat in a woman's health:

Energy Source: Dietary fats are a concentrated source of energy. They provide more than twice the amount of energy per gram compared to carbohydrates and proteins. This stored energy can be used when the body needs additional fuel.

Hormone Production: Fats are essential for the production of hormones, including sex hormones such as estrogen and progesterone. These hormones play critical roles in the menstrual cycle, fertility, and overall reproductive health.

Cell Structure: Fats are a fundamental component of cell membranes. They help maintain the integrity and fluidity of cell membranes, contributing to the proper functioning of cells throughout the body.

Calculating Grams of FAT

<u>Nutrient Absorption:</u> Certain vitamins, such as vitamins A, D, E, and K, are fat-soluble, meaning they need fat for proper absorption. Adequate fat intake ensures the absorption of these essential vitamins, which play roles in bone health, vision, immune function, and antioxidant protection.

<u>Insulation and Temperature Regulation:</u> Adipose tissue, or body fat, serves as insulation, helping to regulate body temperature. It acts as a buffer against temperature changes and provides a protective layer around organs.

<u>Brain Health:</u> The brain is composed of a significant amount of fat, and dietary fats are crucial for brain function. Omega-3 fatty acids, in particular, are essential for cognitive function and are associated with a lower risk of age-related cognitive decline.

<u>Joint Health:</u> Fats play a role in joint lubrication. Omega-3 fatty acids, found in fatty fish and certain plant sources, have anti-inflammatory properties that can benefit joint health.

<u>Skin and Hair Health:</u> Fats contribute to healthy skin and hair. Essential fatty acids, such as omega-6 and omega-3, play a role in maintaining the skin's moisture and elasticity.

It's important to maintain a balanced and varied diet that includes healthy fats, such as those found in avocados, nuts, seeds, olive oil, and fatty fish. At the same time, it's advisable to limit the intake of saturated and trans fats, which are associated with adverse health effects when consumed in excess.

Calculating Grams of FAT

The ideal grams of fat per day for a woman can vary based on factors such as age, activity level, overall health, and individual nutritional needs. However, general dietary guidelines provide a recommended range for daily fat intake as a percentage of total daily caloric intake.

According to the Dietary Guidelines for Americans, the acceptable macronutrient distribution range (AMDR) for fat is:

1. Total Fat: 20% to 35% of total daily caloric intake.

Within this total fat intake:
Saturated Fat: Less than 10% of total daily caloric intake.
Trans Fat: As low as possible.

To determine the ideal grams of fat for a woman on a 2000-calorie per day diet, we can use the recommended percentage range for total fat intake. As mentioned earlier, the acceptable macronutrient distribution range (AMDR) for total fat is 20% to 35% of total daily caloric intake.

Here's how you can calculate it:
Calculate the total fat range:
For a 2000-calorie diet:
Lower limit: 2000 calories x 20% = 400 calories from fat
Upper limit: 2000 calories x 35% = 700 calories from fat

Convert calories from fat to grams:
Since each gram of fat provides 9 calories:
Lower limit: 400 calories / 9 calories per gram = 44.4 grams of fat
Upper limit: 700 calories / 9 calories per gram = 77.7 grams of fat
You can round the number to the nearest whole number for ease.

Calculating Grams of CARBS

Great! So we had 1400 calories left over after calculating our protein goals, and if we take the lower number of ideal fat grams as an example, (44 grams or 400 calories) out of that number, we are left with 1000 calories. This remaining number is what we will calculate our daily carb intake with. Carbohydrates play several crucial roles in a woman's body and nutrition.

Here are some important functions of carbohydrates:

Energy Source: Carbohydrates are the primary and most efficient source of energy for the body. When consumed, carbohydrates are broken down into glucose, which is then used by cells for fuel. This is particularly important for the brain and central nervous system, which rely heavily on glucose for energy.

Metabolic Regulation: Carbohydrates play a role in regulating metabolism. Insulin, a hormone produced by the pancreas, helps regulate blood sugar levels by facilitating the uptake of glucose into cells. This is essential for maintaining stable energy levels and preventing hyperglycemia (high blood sugar) or hypoglycemia (low blood sugar).

Preservation of Lean Body Mass: Adequate carbohydrate intake can help spare protein for its primary functions, such as building and repairing tissues. When there is insufficient carbohydrate intake, the body may use protein for energy, potentially leading to the breakdown of muscle tissue.

Digestive Health: Many carbohydrate-rich foods, such as whole grains, fruits, and vegetables, are excellent sources of dietary fiber. Fiber is essential for maintaining digestive health, promoting regular bowel movements, and preventing constipation. It also contributes to a feeling of fullness and can assist in weight management.

Calculating Grams of CARBS

Supporting Physical Activity: Carbohydrates are a critical energy source during physical activity. Endurance athletes, in particular, rely on stored glycogen (the body's stored form of glucose) to sustain energy during prolonged exercise.

Blood Clotting: Carbohydrates play a role in blood clotting processes. Certain glycoproteins and glycolipids involved in blood clotting contain carbohydrate structures.

Cellular Communication: Carbohydrates are involved in cell signaling and communication. They are components of cell surface receptors, which are crucial for transmitting signals between cells.

Immune System Function: Carbohydrates are involved in immune system function, particularly in the recognition and binding of pathogens by immune cells.

It's important for women to include a variety of carbohydrate sources in their diet, such as whole grains, fruits, vegetables, and legumes. The Dietary Guidelines for Americans recommend that carbohydrates make up 45% to 65% of total daily caloric intake. However, individual needs may vary based on factors such as activity level, age, and overall health.

So back to our math equation. We have 1000 calories remaining, which is 50% of our daily caloric intake- right at the perfect number based on dietary guidelines. And we know that each gram of carbohydrates is 4 calories. So this remaining equation should be very simple!

1000 calories / 4 calories per gram = 250 grams of carbs per day!

How to Create Your Macro Split?
Step 4: Calculate YOUR Goals

Yahoo! We completed our daily macro breakdown for each macronutrient. Let's double check our math!

250 grams of carbs = 1000 calories
44 grams of fat = 396 calories (Rounded up to 400)
150 grams of protein = 600 calories

1000 + 400 + 600 = 2000 calories per day!
Congrats on getting this far! See, it's not as complicated as you might've initially thought. But I needed to include all the details so you have context behind the calculations, and feel confident in your ability to achieve your own caloric goals on your own.

Now I want you to do the math with your own individual numbers below:

__________ grams of protein per day based on weight equals _______ calories
__________ grams of fat per day equals __________ calories
___________ grams of carbohydrates per day equals ___________ calories

I am so proud of you my love! Half the work is done for you now. We can now move onto how to actually track our food in a meal tracking app like MyMacros+ or My Fitness Pal to see how the food you eat breaks down into each gram of macronutrients. You will also find a quick guide to popular whole foods for each macronutrient in a future section if you prefer to do things by hand and not within an app.

How to Create Your Meals?
Step 5: Tracking Food Intake

Calculating macros (macronutrients) using an app like MyFitnessPal or MyMacros+ (my preferred app) involves a few key steps.

Here's a breakdown you can use for your guide:

Step 1: Download and Set Up MyFitnessPal or MyMacros+

Download the app from your app store.
Create an account or log in if you already have one.
Input your personal information like age, gender, weight, height, and activity level if you like. But keep in mind that these apps are not designed to take into consideration your metabolic adaptations like we've calculated. So don't use them as a simple way to calculating your calories. Do that on your own.

Step 2: Set Your Macronutrient Goals

In the app, navigate to the "More" tab (usually located at the bottom right).
Select "Goals" and then choose "Calorie & Macronutrient Goals."
Set your macronutrient goals based on your calculations. This will allow the apps to do the quick math for you when inputting and tracking your foods and meals.

Step 3: Log Your Food Intake

Click on the "+" button to add a food item or find where tracking is located.
Search for the food you are looking to add using the app's extensive database. Many common foods are already entered for quick refence.

How to Create Your Meals?
Step 5: Tracking Food Intake

Enter the quantity or serving size. I always suggest knowing what you have available to eat everyday, or what you are in the mood for, and prepare your meals for the day in the app ahead of time so you're not left with a bunch of random macros to fill at the end of the night, and you can just pull your food and be on the go, instead of obsessing over what to eat. Repeat this process for each food item consumed throughout the day, including all meals and snacks. You will notice each macronutrient number for each individual item as you add it, and see the numbers for your daily goals change. Be mindful to eat to the fulfillment of each number. This is not an option, you need to eat as much as your calories require. Do not limit.

Step 4: Review Your Daily Macronutrient Totals

At the end of the day, go back to the "Diary" tab. Consider if there's anything you snacked on or consumed throughout the day that you forgot to input.

Step 5: Make Adjustments as Needed

If your actual intake is consistently below or above your goals, consider adjusting your food choices to better align with your macronutrient targets.

You can experiment with different food combinations or carb & fat splits to find a balance that works for you while meeting your nutritional needs.

How to Create Your Meals?
Step 5: Tracking Food Intake

Tips:

Use the Barcode Scanner:

These apps allows you to scan barcodes on food packaging for quick and accurate entry. Be sure to cross refence the grams of the serving size on the package to what you are consuming on your own.

Save Frequent Meals:

If you eat similar meals often, you can save them in the app for quicker logging in the future.

Track Beverages and Condiments:

Don't forget to log beverages, cooking oils, and condiments, as they contribute to your daily macronutrient intake. This is where many people fall off the deep end, as condiments like salad dressings, coffee creamers, and things along those lines add more calories than you may realize and they add up awfully fast. It may seem tedious, but adding 300 calories worth of 3 tablespoons of caesar dressing is important, especially when you're unsure why you aren't losing fat when you believe you've been eating on plan.

Remember, while tracking macros can be a useful tool, it's essential to prioritize overall health and well-being. Individual nutritional needs vary, and it's advisable to consult with a healthcare professional or a registered dietitian for personalized guidance if you're unsure of what to do.

How to Know When to Change?
Step 6: Evolving Your Goals

You are killing this guide!

Okay, now a final piece of this puzzle is assessing your progress and knowing when it's time to evolve your goals and meals so you continue progressing.

You started off in a recomp phase and most women can stay there for quite some time and continue to see progress. But as I mentioned in the very beginning, eventually your body adapts. Now, adapting to a higher caloric intake and maintaining an ideal body composition is a great thing, yes, but what if you realize that your goal is to finally enter a gaining phase to add on more muscle tissue? Or, what if after you've fixed your metabolic issues you want to actually attempt a real fat loss phase? Well then it means we need to take our recomp calories and either add to them, or subtract from them.

There are some easy ways to do this, but remember that after you've gotten your body used to a certain caloric intake number, when we decide to drop or raise calories, the body will change based on that new goal, and with changes always come fluctuations, so don't expect this process to ever be totally linear. It's normal and natural.

As mentioned in the beginning of the guide,
3500 calories = 1 pound

The same is true for adding muscle tissue or losing fat, however adding a pound of quality muscle tissue is harder to do than losing a pound of body fat.

How to Know When to Change?
Step 6: Evolving Your Goals

So, if after you've gotten through some consistent time in a recomp phase and you want to start a fat loss phase, we are going to have to consider how quickly we want to lose this weight and over how long. The following is a method of going about this so long as everything is working optimally to begin with. Any resistance to fat loss may be due to hormonal, thyroid, or other health issues so please be sure to get bloodwork periodically to ensure all your levels are optimal for a fat loss phase.

I also mentioned previously that the goal is never to lose more than 1-2 pounds per week, because beyond that you are going to encounter health and metabolic problems and wind yourself back in the same place you were before you started. Let's be sure not to backtrack and only evolve forwards.

So say a good goal is to lose 10 pounds over 10 weeks, 1 pound per week. Realize that losing weight is not the same as losing fat. So that is where your previous experiene of tracking all points of data like weight, measurements, and progress photos will come into play.

But for purposes of ease in learning, we will keep things simple.
3500 calories over the course of 7 days = -500 calories per day.

For an example, if your daily calories started at 2000 per day in your recomp phase, we will have to subtract 500 calories per day to start this fat loss phase, giving you 1500 calories per day. A rule of thumb is the longer you want to diet, the less of a caloric drop you want to have per day, or you start dipping into dangerous waters. This is also relative to your daily intake. If your daily TDEE is not 2000 calories per day or more, you must be very careful to do this slowly and over time.

How to Know When to Change?
Step 6: Evolving Your Goals

To create your fat loss calories and macros of 1500 per day, you want to be sure to keep these things in mind, as they are of utmost importance:

- Keep your protein intake where it has been, or at the lowest, at your anticipated goal weight. So if you are looking to lose 10lbs, the most you want to remove is 10g of protein per day.

- If you are someone who has pulled their fat grams goal from the lower end of the spectrum, the majority of your calories should be taken from your carbohydrates.

- If you are someone who has pulled their fat grams goals from the higher end of the spectrum, start by pulling back your fat grams until they reach a moderate level, and pull the remaining calories from your carbs until you achieve your ideal caloric number.

The same is true for those of you who are looking to gain weight and/or lean muscle tissue. Gaining muscle is a harder process and takes a bit more time for women, but it is possible with a good and consistent plan.

If you are looking to simply gain weight, and don't care about whether that weight is fat or muscle, then you want to reverse the process and instead of subtracting 500 calories per day like you would in the fat loss phase, you will be adding 500 calories per day. These 500 calories should be added in the form of fats and carbs predominantly, and keep protein the same.

However, if you are looking to add quality muscle tissue, you will want to be a bit more meticulous with this process.

How to Know When to Change?
Step 6: Evolving Your Goals

Giving yourself time to grow is important when the goal is muscle.

So let's start by adding 500 calories per day, in hopes of adding a pound per week. As mentioned previously, that weight that you gain will not be ALL muscle or ALL fat. As long as you are strength training consistently, and advancing with your weights in the gym, you will gain muscle. Your protein should remain at 1 gram per pound of body weight, but adding 5-10 grams per day over the course of 2-3 months is ideal.

Within the 500 calorie addition, you also want to increase your carbs and fats periodically. Increasing carbs first is most beneficial to muscle gain, as carbs help energize the muscle and keep glycogen fueling its gains and recovery.

Fats are also important for digestion of the carbs, but I've found that keeping fats at an optional level for health, within that 20%-35% range is ideal. There are less muscle building properties in fats than there are in carbs, which is why we want to keep fats in a range that is optimal for health and digestion, but increase carbohydrates over time to ensure they are facilitating muscle growth, but not facilitating fat gain.

As long as you are consistent with your meals and training, you will gain muscle. Give yourself some months in a gaining phase, and when you believe you have reached an ideal muscular level for your goals, you can then start to cut back the food and possibly enter a short fat loss phase to reveal what you have built during that time, and show the true development of the muscle against the skin, as we do as bodybuilders and competitors.

Remember to have fun and allow yourself to grow more than just physically!

Non Fitness Goals

Jot down your current NON PHYSICAL long & short term goals.

Family/Friends/Social

Financial/Career

Hobby/Interest/Dream

Notes:

Your Tools & Resources

Use this portion as a reference point for tools, items, and apps
to compile your data to stay on track!

FOOD RELATED:

- ☐ MyFitnessPal or MyMacros+
- ☐ Food Scale
- ☐ Body Weight Scale
- ☐ Tape Measurer

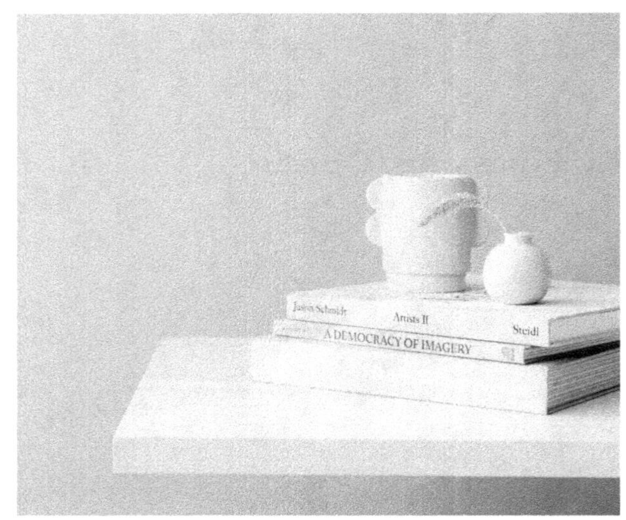

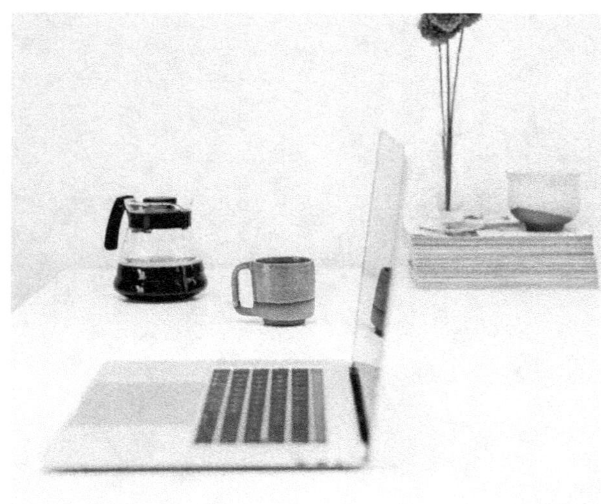

FITNESS RELATED:

- ☐ Workout Program
- ☐ Gym Membership
- ☐ Foam Roller
- ☐ Resistance Bands
- ☐ Good Sneakers

Goal Macros:

1900 Calories
140g Protein - 560 cals
200g Carbs - 800 cals
60g Fat - 540 cals

Daily Meal Plan Example

Take the time today to test your tracking and plug these foods into your MyFitnessPal app. I want you to get the hang of creating a meal, and filling in the amount of each item to help reach your goals. If there are items you hate included in the example meal, try swapping it out with one of the alternatives and see what you can create and make work! You want to get within 10g MAX of each macronutrient at the end of the day.

BREAKFAST

4 Large Egg Whites, 1 Whole Egg, 40g Quick Oats, 60g Banana, 16g Peanut Butter

Total Macros:

29.9g Protein | 45.3g Carbs | 15.9g Fat | 441.5 Calories

LUNCH

3.5oz Chicken Breast, 3oz Sweet Potato (or 150g red potato)
2oz Avocado, 12g Salted Almonds

Total Macros:

35.7g Protein | 30.8g Carbs | 16.4g Fat | 399 Calories

DINNER

4oz 93/7% Lean Ground Turkey, 100g COOKED Jasmine/White Rice, 85g Green Vegetable, 1 Herb & Garlic Laughing Cow Cheese Triangle

Total Macros:

28.2g Protein | 33.4g Carbs | 9.5g Fat | 334.8 Calories

SNACK

35g PEScience Chocolate Cupcake Whey Protein Powder (or 1 Scoop Protein Powder of Your Choice) 290mL Fat Free Milk, 16g Smooth Peanut Butter, Ice to Blend, 2 Apple Cinnamon Rice Cakes, 1 Caramel Rice Cake, 18g Peanut Butter to spread. 2 Rice Krispy Treats.

Total Macros:

45.9g Protein | 91.2g Carbs | 22.6g Fat | 757.6 Calories

Macro Totals:

1933 Calories | 139.7g Protein | 200.7g Carbs | 64.3g Fat

Food Shopping List

Below you'll find a list of popular foods to incorporate within your weekly shopping list. It's your responsibility to fill your macros with the foods that you enjoy and will get you closer to your goals. You will see a combination of healthy, whole foods combined with some processed options.

Protein Sources (Animal & Plant Based)

- Chicken Breast
- Ground Turkey (85-99% lean)
- Ground Beef (85-97%)
- Eggs/Egg Whites
- Cod
- Steak
- Lamb
- Black Beans
- Bison
- Lentils
- Tempeh
- Tofu
- Chickpea Pasta
- Tuna
- Salmon
- Tilapia
- Pork
- Whey Protein
- Seitan
- Veal
- Pea Protein
- Greek Yogurt

Food Shopping List

Full Carb Sources & Low Carb Vegetable Sources

- Butternut Squash
- Cantaloupe
- Pineapple
- Bananas
- Rice Cakes
- Potatoes
- Sweet Potato/Yams
- Assorted Rices
- Quinoa
- Oatmeal
- Apples
- Oranges
- Corn
- Vegetables
- Cereal
- Cream of Rice
- Cream of Wheat
- Pasta
- Bread
- English Muffins
- Berries
- Grits
- Tortillas
- Beans
- Honey
- Buckwheat
- Barley
- Hummus
- Granola
- Spinach
- Kale
- Asparagus
- Mushrooms
- Cauliflower
- Peppers
- Leeks
- Lettuce
- Snow Peas
- Zucchini
- Carrots
- Peas & Carrots Mix
- Arugula
- Alfalfa Sprouts
- Kohlrabi
- Cabbage
- Eggplant
- Onions
- Seaweed
- Broccoli
- Brussel Sprouts
- Celery
- Cucumber
- Green Beans
- Okra
- Turnips
- Beets
- Radish
- Chard
- Broccoli Rabe
- Tomatoes

Food Shopping List

Fat Sources

- Pumpkin Seeds
- Cashews
- Cashew Butter
- Avocado
- Avocado Oil
- Coconut Oil
- Hazelnuts
- Almond Butter
- Chia Seeds
- Walnut Oil
- Almonds
- Sesame Oil
- Pecans
- Walnuts
- Butter
- Pistachios
- Coconut Butter
- Brazil Nuts
- Olives
- Olive Oil
- Macadamias
- Peanut Butter
- Peanuts
- Flaxseeds
- Flaxseed Oil
- Vegetable Oil
- Canola Oil
- Egg Yolks
- Cheeses
- Dark Chocolate

Food Shopping List

Condiments & Additives

- Splenda
- Stevia
- Sweet & Low
- Equal
- Cinnamon
- Mrs. Dash Seasonings
- Sea Salt
- White Table Salt
- Pepper
- Fat Free Pan Spray
- "I Can't Believe It's Not Butter" Spray/Spread
- Pasta Sauce
- Sugar Free Pancake Syrup
- Low Sugar Heinz Ketchup
- Parmesan Cheese
- Half & Half
- Low Fat Milk
- 1% Milk
- 2% Milk
- Whole Milk
- Almond Milk
- Cashew Milk
- Oat Milk
- Mustard
- G. Hughes Honey Mustard
- G. Hughes BBQ Sauce
- G. Hughes Teriyaki Sauce
- Laughing Cow Cheese Spreads

Macro Swap Cheat Sheet

Below you'll find the quick macros for some popular foods. It's your responsibility to fill your macros with the foods that you enjoy and will get you closer to your goals. You may have to manipulate the portions to hit your macros exactly, so utilize MyFitnessPal to calculate for you.

Protein Based Carb Based Fat Based	Size & Calories	Protein	Carbs	Fats
Chicken Breast	4oz/147 cal	**34g**	**0g**	**1.2g**
93/7 Lean Ground Turkey	4oz/160 cal	**22g**	**0g**	**8g**
Large Egg White	17 Cal	**3.6g**	**0g**	**0.1g**
Liquid Egg Whites	46g/25 cal	**0g**	**1g**	**5g**
92% Lean Beef	4oz/165 cal	**21g**	**0g**	**9g**
96% Lean Beef	4oz/140 cal	**24g**	**0g**	**5g**
Salmon Wild Alaska	4oz/173 cal	**29.3g**	**0g**	**5.3g**
Tilapia	4oz/110 cal	**21g**	**0g**	**2g**
Cod Fish	4oz/96 cal	**20g**	**0g**	**0.8g**
Shrimp	4oz/91 cal	**22.7g**	**0g**	**0g**

Macro Swap Cheat Sheet

Below you'll find the quick macros for some popular foods. It's your responsibility to fill your macros with the foods that you enjoy and will get you closer to your goals. You may have to manipulate the portions to hit your macros exactly, so utilize MyFitnessPal to calculate for you.

Protein Based

Carb Based

Fat Based

	Size & Calories	Protein	Carbs	Fats
Albacore Tuna	4oz/120 cal	26g	0g	2g
99% Lean Ground Turkey	4oz/120 cal	28g	0g	1g
Sweet Potatoes	4oz/104 cal	2.4g	23.6g	0.1g
White Potatoes	100g/87 cal	2.2g	20.4g	0.1g
Red Potatoes	4oz/110 cal	3g	26g	0g
Brown Rice	45g Dry/170cal	4g	35g	1g
Jasmine Rice	45g dry/160 cal	3g	36g	0.5g
Quick Oats	50g dry/188 cal	6.2g	33.8g	3.1g
Banana	100g/57 cal	0g	14.3g	0g
Blueberries	100g/47 cal	0g	11.8g	0g

Macro Swap Cheat Sheet

Below you'll find the quick macros for some popular foods. It's your responsibility to fill your macros with the foods that you enjoy and will get you closer to your goals. You may have to manipulate the portions to hit your macros exactly, so utilize MyFitnessPal to calculate for you.

	Size & Calories	Protein	Carbs	Fats
Strawberries	100g/34 cal	0.7g	7.9g	0g
Avocado	55g/96 cal	1g	4.8g	8.7g
Smooth Peanut Butter	16g/94 cal	3.8g	3.5g	8g
Half & Half	16g/18 cal	0.5g	0.5g	1.5g
Olive Oil	15g/126 cal	0g	0g	14g
Coconut Oil	15g/120 cal	0g	0g	14g
Whole Milk	250ml/160 cal	8g	13g	8g
Mexican Shredded Cheese Blend	28g/110 cal	6g	1g	8g
Almonds	15g/90 cal	3g	3g	8g
Egg Whole	69 cal	6g	0g	5g

Your Main Food Sources

The goal of this page is to list out the food sources for each macronutrient that you believe you'd be able to have prepared and ready to eat regularly. Meal prep is half the battle.

Protein Sources

Carbohydrate Sources

Fat Sources

Thank you!

i want to let you know just how appreciative I am of you purchasing this guide and supporting me. I hope you got everything you were looking to learn out of this, and I want to know how it works out for you!

Feel free to send me a message anytime to let me know about your progress and results from following this guide and flexible dieting, and feel free to reach out with any questions along the way!

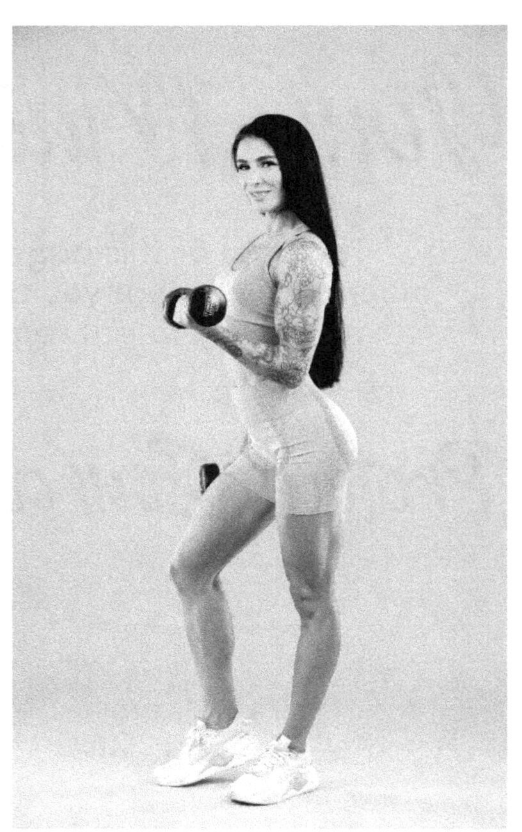

Do You Want More Help?

Send me a message or email!
@christinaifbbpro on Instagram
info.christinafriscia@gmail.com

Looking to work together 1:1 to reach your fitness and physique goals? Fill out my coaching application and you'll receive a custom video going over my feedback & critiques as well as the info to get started on coaching!